Healthy after 55

Live Your Best Life

Simple Steps to Help Women Regain and Maintain Their Health

Julie Luedtke

DISCLAIMER

The information provided in this book is for educational purposes only. I am not a doctor and this is not meant to be taken as medical advice. The information provided in this guide is based on my experiences as well as my interpretation of the current research available.

The advice and tips given are meant for healthy adults only. Please consult your physician to ensure the tips given in the book are appropriate for your individual circumstances.

If you have any health issues or pre-existing conditions, please consult with your physical before implementing any of the information provided in this book.

This book is for informational purposes only and the author does not accept any responsibilities for any liabilities or damages, real or perceived, resulting from the use of this information.

I would like to dedicate this book to the following people:

My children, Kari, Bonnie and Scot have encouraged me to write this book and share what I have learned to help other women. They have been my chief cheerleaders, kept me grounded, and surrounded me with their love.

My accountability buddy, Ann, kept me on track. She gave me great advice on content and editing, and we shared a lot of laughs along the way.

Ramy, my coach at Self-Publishing School, shared so much information to help me make this book the best it could be. With his help, I avoided the dreaded procrastination and met my goals.

My fitness classes for women over 55 who encouraged me to share the skills and ideas that have helped them live their best life.

CONTENTS

Introduction

What have you done for yourself lately?

Your life revolved around children, spouse, career, and a hundred details that kept you busy every day. No time to think about yourself. You were busy taking care of everyone else.

Now it's different. You have reached an age where your children have left home, you may or may not have a spouse, and your career is stable.

You think about interests you didn't have time to pursue years ago. You are restless. You look up at a flight of steps … then search for the elevator because you just don't think you can make it to the second floor.

Is it too late to start a new life or follow your passion? Absolutely not!

What makes this book different from all the other health and wellness books on the market? *This book was created by someone who learned by trial and error to live these steps every day, and continues to do so 20 years later.*

I guarantee this book will help you take the steps necessary to lead a life that is not only healthy, but happy and fulfilling.

You deserve to be confident about taking care of yourself and maintaining your independence. This book helps you take the first steps toward the next phase in your life's journey. The journey you earned and deserve.

My Story: I Learned These Lessions the Hard Way

As I made my way through my 40s and 50s I can't tell you how many dead-end roads I traveled …and had to turn around and try again. That's why I decided to write this book to save you the wasted time, energy and expense.

That is how the first steps of my journey to health and wellness began …and it is the inspiration for this book.

I read books and did as much research as possible …before the ease of using Google search. I started to walk and then run.

I even did a 5k race (very slowly). I took a spin class at the gym, I cleaned out my refrigerator and pantry …and sadly said "good-bye" to my chocolate ice cream (it was an empty carton by the time I finished my "good-bye").

It wasn't easy. Many days were a huge challenge, but I continued to take one step at a time to regain my health and be happy again.

And where did this crazy journey take me?

Slowly I began to see a healthy, positive future.

I did my first marathon …yes, all 26.2 miles on foot at the age of 55, started *teaching* the spin class where I took my first class, and did a 100-mile bike ride at 57. I thought this part of my journey was complete.

It was just beginning.

As I write this book, I'm 73 and retired from corporate life. I have done multiple 100-mile bike rides, sprint triathlons, completed four marathons, more half marathons than I can remember as well as 10k and 5k races that are a blur (not because I was so fast, but because there have been so many of them). I have no plans to stop competing.

An important part of my journey is to continue to help other older adults live a healthy, vibrant, active life … *and I can help you, too.*

As a certified personal trainer and certified to train older adults, I incorporate the steps in this book in exercise classes I teach. Participants increased their health and happiness. And, yes, those participants are the inspiration for this book as well as a focus group for what works and what doesn't.

You've probably tried many ways to be healthy …

How is it working for you so far?

If it was easy to be healthy by just following a diet and doing some exercise every day, you wouldn't be reading this book!

You start a healthy program, fall off the wagon, shake your head, and go back to unhealthy habits. Then a few months later, start all over again.

I am going to show you in just *three minutes* how important reading this book is to the quality of your life, and how you can continue to live a healthy lifestyle every day.

Sit in a comfortable chair without any distractions. Read the first step and then close your eyes and imagine yourself in that position.

Scene 1: You are sitting on the floor playing with your grandchild. There is a gust of wind, the door flies open and your grandchild runs toward the open door and toward the street. You are unable to get to your feet quickly, and you call out to your grandchild, but they don't listen to you. They are outside and headed for the street before you can reach them. How do you feel?

Now, after you think about that, read Scene 2 and imagine yourself in a little different scenario.

Scene 2: You are sitting on the floor playing with your grandchild. There is a gust of wind, the door flies open and your grandchild runs toward the open door and toward the street. You scramble to your feet and rush to grab your precious grandchild before they are injured. You are filled with gratitude that you were able to react quickly.

Can you see what a difference this one incident would make if you were healthy?

Now, you understand the importance of this book. This is the reason it is vital to take the first step for a healthy, vibrant future.

If you decide not to read this book, how will you take the steps necessary to regain your health? Keep trying different diets? Join the gym, but don't go? I've been there, done that.

Read this book and follow the simple steps for a life-time of health.

Participants in my classes have been where I was and where you are right now. The difference? They took those first steps to gain control of their lives and be healthier and happier. You can do the same thing …in the comfort of your own home.

My goal is to help _you_ increase the _quality_ of your life. _Quality_ of life becomes even more important as we get older. You want to maintain your independence with each passing year.

If you are 55 right now, you could easily live another 30 or more years. Think of what you can accomplish in that time if you are healthy and enthusiastic about life …or you can sit in a chair, watch TV, and accomplish nothing.

I will take you through easy-to-follow steps to make your life happier and healthier. Start _today_ on this important journey.

Laura, one of my students, said, "I wasn't sure about life after retirement. A friend had to drag me to your class the first time. I had a pocket full of excuses. But she talked me into coming to your class. By taking your class and following your steps, I have renewed confidence, enjoy playing with my grandchildren, and really enjoy retirement."

I promise that if you read my book, take that first step and continue on the journey, you will feel better, have more energy and a renewed zest for life.

Don't be the person who sighs and murmurs, "Maybe tomorrow or next year." Be the person who takes charge of their life and becomes an inspiration.

The time you invest in reading this book and taking the steps to increase the quality of your life is minimal compared to the benefits you will receive for years to come.

The theme of this book is **J.O.Y. = Just One Yes.**

Every day that you do something good for yourself — from taking a walk to meditating, give yourself a pat on the back for **J.O.Y.**

Health is your first wealth!

Chapter #1
Reality Check

How to define what is important in your life

THIS IS A REALITY CHECK. STOP AVOIDING the mirror and pretending you look like the model on a cover of a magazine.

In this chapter, you will discover what is really important in your life and how to maintain your health as you continue moving forward.

Let's face it…reality sucks. I can close my eyes and see myself at 30, slim and trim, full of life and enthusiasm. Then I open my eyes, look in the mirror and just shake my head. Gravity is just plain mean.

Reality can be a positive factor as well. You can find all kinds of things to be grateful for after all these years …maybe additions to your family, the time to take vacations, your ability to see a beautiful sunrise or sunset, the time to read a favorite book.

Starting the journey may be the most difficult part. Beginning another diet is depressing. Going out the door for a walk is daunting. Sometimes it's easier to sit in your favorite chair with a bowl of ice cream and watch your favorite show.

Your First Challenge.

Close your eyes and remember how you felt when you imagined that you couldn't get off the floor to save your grandchild. Is that how you want to feel for the rest of your life? Of course not.

Since this is a reality check, I want you to understand that it won't always be easy and sometimes, it won't be much fun. But if you continue to move toward your goal, the rewards are worth the effort.

Think about what you realistically want your life to be …then realize that not only do you *want* it, but it is necessary for the *quality* of your life.

WARNING: If you choose to take this challenge, you will feel better, be happier and healthier. You will have the strength to get up off the floor by yourself. Maybe your old clothes will fit again and the next time you go to the doctor, you will look forward to getting your blood pressure checked. It could happen … and it *will* happen, but you need to take the first step.

Each chapter in this book has a unique way for you to set your goals. The goal for this first chapter and continuing through the book is **J.O.Y. = Just One Yes**.

Every day do something positive for yourself. This is the time to be selfish. Think about something positive you've done for yourself, raise your arms in the air, and say, "YES!" It can be anything from taking a walk to eating a piece of fruit instead of a candy bar.

Every positive thing you do for yourself is **J.O.Y.**

So … are you ready for *your* reality check and your first challenge? Are you ready to spread some J.O.Y. in your life?

Start today … it's *your* life and *your* choice.

On the next page is a checklist to get you thinking about *your* reality. Be honest. This is for you and about you. Think of this as your homework for the next three months.

There are five questions in each category.

- Print the checklist and keep it where you will see it every day ... the bathroom mirror or the refrigerator.

- Every day, look at the list and make a plan to change just one thing.

- Every week, change one "No" into a "*Yes*".

Your Motivation to Accomplish Health and Wellness

Start date	One month "Yes"	Two months "Yes"	Three months "Yes"
___________	___________	___________	___________

Kitchen

Yes No

☐ ☐ Look in your refrigerator. Are there healthy choices at eye level?

☐ ☐ Are there *any* healthy foods in your refrigerator?

☐ ☐ Look in your pantry. Are there healthy choices?

☐ ☐ Do you drink at least eight glasses of water every day?

☐ ☐ Do you track the food/calories you eat every day?

Closet

Yes   No

☐ ☐ Can you wear any of the clothes you wore two years ago?

☐ ☐ Do you have a favorite outfit in your closet that you want to wear, but can't fit into?

☐ ☐ Can you zip and button your pants that don't have elastic in the waist?

☐ ☐ Have you gone shopping for clothes in the last six months because you *wanted to* instead of the need to find something that fits?

☐ ☐ Do you wear black all the time because it makes you look slim?

Fitness

Yes   No

☐ ☐ Can you bend over and touch your feet?

☐ ☐ Can you pick up a bag of groceries and carry it into the house without getting out of breath?

☐ ☐ Do you wake up in the morning energetic and ready to face the day?

☐ ☐ Have you taken a walk in the last week?

☐ ☐ If you fell down, would you be able to get up?

Socialization/Attitude

Yes　No

☐ ☐ Have you made an effort to sit down and talk to a friend without any distractions in the last two months?

☐ ☐ Have you banished the excuse that you are "too old" to do something?

☐ ☐ Did you set goals a month ago that you continue to keep?

☐ ☐ Are you passionate about your effort to be healthy?

☐ ☐ Do you smile when you look in the mirror?

One or less "Yes" in each category, you really need to read every chapter of this book as soon as possible.

Two "Yes" in each category, you are making progress, but need to have a plan to make more progress.

Three "Yes" checkmarks in each category and you are making progress. J.O.Y. is on the horizon.

Four "Yes" check marks and you are a star! Give yourself a pat on the back and work on those last few check marks.

All "Yes" check marks and you are a Super Star! Keep up the good work and read on …

NOTE: You can download a pdf or print all the homework pages at our website www.HealthyAfter55.com

The Challenge is Real

When I started my wellness journey, I might have had a couple of "yes" check marks. I could almost touch my toes. That should count for something. And I looked in the mirror with a smirk on my face. That was almost a "yes".

I started where you are today and I'm on that journey for the rest of my life. Some days are great. I am positive I have conquered the mountain.

Then there are days I just have to shake my head, take a deep breath, and plod on. But, I'm here to tell you, *it is worth the effort.*

It's time to enjoy the life you've earned.

Quality of life and your health are priceless!

This chapter is about doing a reality check. The checklist you just started puts this journey into perspective. Let's face it. For most of our adult lives, women put someone else's needs before their own. We are girlfriends, wives, mothers, employees, employers, chief cook, queen of grocery shopping, etc.

It's not easy to put ourselves first. We grew up thinking that is was selfish (bad) to think about ourselves before others. This may take some time for you to embrace the feeling, but once you do, you will realize that it's not selfish.

When you take time for yourself, you enhance your relationship with everyone around you. When you take care of your own needs first, you have more energy and health to take care of others.

Will this make you happier? It's amazing what a difference these first steps will make for your own peace of mind.

Laughter is a Healthy Start

Recent studies have shown that even if you are not feeling very happy, fake laughter works just like real laughter on your mind and body. When participants were instructed to laugh out loud, even if it was a fake laugh, their endorphins increased, blood flow was stimulated and it started the process of genuine laughter.

When participants exercised, it was with a little more intensity and the laughter increased the benefits of the exercise. Who knew laughter would benefit exercise and your health?

I tried this with one of my exercise classes. One morning they were just going through the motions of exercising. I stopped the class and asked them to start laughing for 30 seconds … big belly laughs. At first they just giggled, but as I encouraged them, they actually started to smile and laugh. When they returned to exercising, they had renewed energy.

Stop reading this book for just 30 seconds and laugh. It sounds fake when you begin, but soon you will smile and really laugh.

Congratulations! You just accomplished your first **J.O.Y.**

Motivation to Begin Your Journey of J.O.Y.

Start to turn those "No" checkmarks on your reality checklist to a "Yes".

1. Close your eyes and think of how far you've come in life's journey. Take a deep breath through your nose, exhale through your mouth and focus for a minute on where you started as an adult and where you are now. Think about your priorities then … and now. How has life changed for you? Think about what you would like to change.

2. Start with one small step. Restore **J.O.Y.** and add **zest** to your life through gratitude. Use a small notebook, and when you wake up in the morning or before you go to sleep at night, write down something you are grateful for that day. This simple act can have a positive effect on your body and mind.

3. Do something that brings you **J.O.Y.** …work in your garden, bake, read, knit, build something, play with your grandchild or pet …whatever makes you happy.

4. If you could do *one* thing that you always wanted to do, but put it off for any number of reasons, what would it be? Take piano lessons? Learn to play the guitar?

5. Perhaps you always wanted a pet, but you were too busy, traveled for work, just didn't do it. Adopt an animal. Cats and dogs are guaranteed to make you smile and give you **J.O.Y.** Not only will you help an animal find a new home, but you will be more active and enjoy the companionship. A win-win for everyone involved.

My neighbor retired a couple of years ago and had trouble adjusting to her new lifestyle. After several months, she adopted a rescue dog. Tammy said, "This dog has made a huge difference in my life and my outlook on retirement. I get outside every day to go for a walk, interact with other people in the neighborhood, and have a new zest for life." **Note**: She suggests adopting an older cat or dog rather than a puppy or kitten. They are already trained and not so energetic.

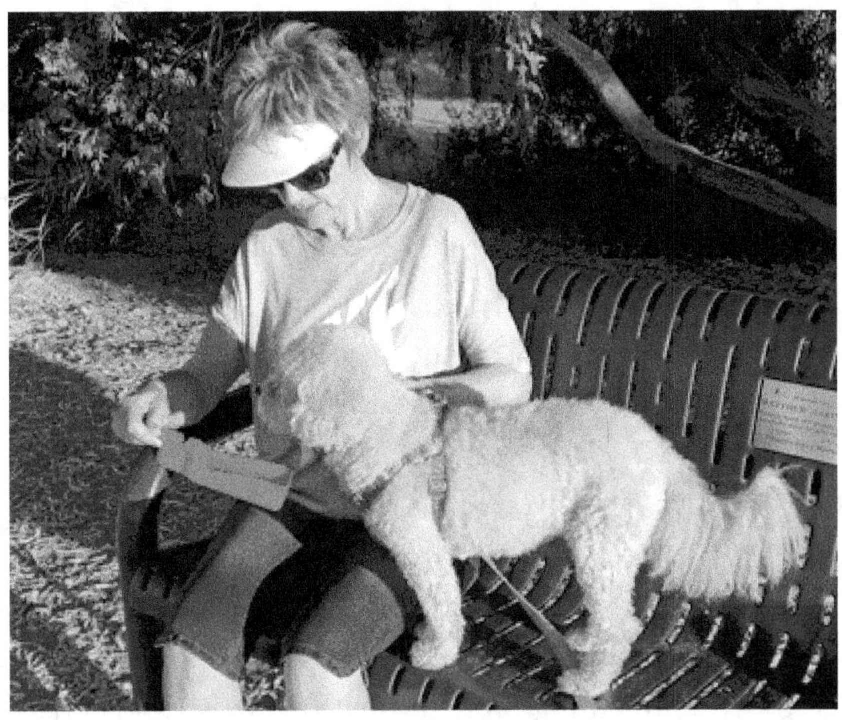

In this chapter we discussed different ways to create **J.O.Y** in your life. It may feel overwhelming at first, but take it one small step at a time.

Use your checklist as a daily reminder of steps to take to regain your health.

Sara's Story

Sara is a woman I helped a couple of years ago. Sara was in her 60s and diagnosed with a brain tumor. She had surgery, but became very depressed.

Her daughter knew that I was a personal trainer for adults over the age of 55 and asked me to help her mother regain her strength. The first time I met Sara, she was frail, shuffled her feet, wouldn't look at me, and wore a scarf over her head to hide the scar.

Whenever I work with someone, I evaluate their physical, mental, and emotional abilities so I know how to start a program that is specific for them. When I shook her hand, she had a very firm handshake. That was a good sign.

The first thing we did was create her personal J.O.Y. journal. She had a big calendar, so every day between our sessions, she had to write something on that calendar that she was grateful for. It became a focal point for her and her family to see the progress on that calendar.

You will hear more of Sara's story through the following chapters. Sara will inspire you to set your goals and accomplish the J.O.Y. in your life.

The reality checklist puts your health into perspective.

There are simple ways to bring back the J.O.Y. in your life and they are doable, no matter how busy you are.

When I started the journey to restore my health, there wasn't a lot of information for women over the age of 50. No one discussed menopause and the effect it had on not only your body, but your mind, attitude and life in general.

I learned through trial and lots of errors what worked, what was a waste of time, and what was just hilarious. I will share some of those stories in our quest to reach the mountain top.

What you learned in this chapter to feel J.O.Y.

- Just One Yes for yourself every day

- Start with one small step

- Do something that gives you pleasure

- After years of nurturing others, become aware of *your* health

- Try something new that you always wanted to do, but never had the time

- If not now ... when?

The next chapter will help you take the first steps toward regaining your health. Your health is a work in progress, so take these steps in order, one at a time. Remember, the effort you put into each step will help you move toward the next step and the next goal.

Now, it's time to take the first step.

NOTE: Whenever I work with an individual as a personal trainer, or in a class setting, I always make sure that the participants have checked with their health care professional. I ask them to share with me what their health care professional told them regarding what they should be doing to increase their health and what they should avoid to prevent injury.

Nothing in this book should be considered medical advice. Always consult a doctor before making any changes to your diet, medical plan, exercise routine, or anything else that is important to your health. Be informed and make the best decision for your health!

Chapter #2
Get Started

How to Take the First Step

Now it's time to get started toward your goal of a healthier, happier life. By the time you complete this chapter, you will begin to move forward.

Many of you used S.M.A.R.T. goals in your business life. I've simplified the system of setting goals to make acronyms relevant for this journey.

Our first acronym is **J.O.Y.** We talked about it in the last chapter. Now we are going to use it.

J is for Just
O is for One
Y is for Yes

To begin the process, sit down where you can think without distractions. Grab a pencil and a notebook so you can take the time to write down your answers. Turn off the television, cell phone, and computer. Take a few deep breaths and relax.

The homework for this chapter may seem simple, but take the time to answer every question honestly.

Print out this worksheet. You are the only one who will see the answers, so let your mind wander.

Write your answers in the space provided.

Look at your answers while you read this book. Maybe you will modify some of them, or change them completely, but take the step forward.

Homework for this chapter about J.O.Y.

The JOY in Setting Goals

1. *What would you like to accomplish during this chapter of your life?* You are over the age of 55, but your life is not over. You could live for another 30 or 40 years. Think about that. You have time to accomplish so much that has been pushed aside while your life moved through career and family responsibilities. Now you have time for yourself.

2. *What are two things you have experienced through the years that you could share with others that might make an impact on their lives?* Take a moment to think about what you've accomplished and what you have to share. It could be something to do with balancing a career and motherhood. It could be the importance of deciding whether to get married and have children or stay single.

First experience:

Second experience:

3. *What are three things you want to be able to do 20 years from now?* Age is a state of mind. Take stock of your physical, mental and emotional health. Have you said to yourself or others, "I'm too old to do that"? Think about the things that would be important for you in the future and how you want to feel at that age. It could involve increased energy, eating healthy meals on a consistent basis, the ability to climb a flight of steps without huffing and puffing, or watching your grandchildren graduate from high school or college.

First goal:

Second goal:

Third goal:

4. *What will you never wear again that is stashed in your closet?* Go through your entire closet and be realistic. If it has been more than six months since you've tried something on, take the time and try on every item. Look in the mirror while you struggle to put them on. Separate them into three piles. Pile #1 actually fits and you would wear them in public, pile #2 is "someday I'll fit in them again" and pile #3 is "never again." Ask yourself how many of the clothes in pile #2 need to be moved to pile #3 … and donate them to charity.

Write down five items in your closet that you want to wear in the next six months, then move them to the front of your closet and try them on every month until they fit.

5. *What would you love to do if you had the time, energy and resources to do it?* Let your imagination soar. You probably had a passion for something when you were younger, but life got in the way. Close your eyes and think about what you would do. Nothing is off limits.

Five simple questions ... but your answers will not only open your eyes to your life right now, but also how you would like to live for years to come.

The choice is yours. You can sit and wonder what might have been or open up to exciting adventures.

As you embark on this journey, remember the JOY you found in your youth. Use those memories to focus on the adventures to come.

NOTE: You can download a pdf or print all the homework pages at our website www.HealthyAfter55.com

Start the Journey Forward by Going Back in Time

After answering the five questions, take time to write about your family history or reminisce about family adventures that you enjoyed. Think about the years when you were growing up. What gave you pleasure? What was your favorite toy? Did you go on vacations? Did you have pets? Were there special holidays?

Think about your answer to question #5. Start with that passion. You may modify it, or change it completely, but it's a place to start. See if that passion ignites a new flame or makes you smile as you find something else that lights a fire within you.

Incentive for grumpy woman to get strong...

When I was doing personal training at a local health club some years ago, I worked with a woman in her early 70s who had fallen down and was in need of strength training. She was grumpy and her first words to me were, "My kids made me come here and do this. I'm old. What difference will some silly exercises make?"

Before I set up a plan for her, we talked. My first question to her was, "Your children are obviously concerned about you. They care. Why do you think they want you to be strong?"

She started to talk about falling down and her fear of losing her independence. She was very honest. "I love my children, but I don't want to live with them and they don't want me to live with them. It would drive all of us crazy. And I don't want to end up in a home with a bunch of old buzzards." *That* was her incentive to get strong.

We worked together every week. I gave her simple things she could do at home if the weather prevented her from getting to the gym. Over two months of working together, her attitude improved. She actually smiled when she showed me that she could get down on the floor and stand up without any help. Her grip had improved and she started to make jewelry again. She gave me an impish grin when she told me that she went out for breakfast with a gentleman she met at the gym.

Just two months and she was making positive changes in her life. It just took a nudge from her children. And yes, she begrudgingly said she appreciated what they had done to give her that initial push toward better health.

Here are some ideas that might give you a nudge to accomplish your goals.

1. Pull out an old photo of yourself when you were young, happy, and looking forward to life with enthusiasm. Put that picture where you can see it every day and smile. It's not too late to regain that feeling … and enhance it with the wisdom you've gained through the years.

2. Resist the urge to compare yourself and your life at this time to anyone else. Everyone has a different story. ***You are unique; enjoy this exciting path of your life's journey.***

3. Think about a favorite memory and everything that surrounded it. What were you doing and how did you feel? Does that memory stir some new interests?

Stay in the present moment … you can't do anything about the past or the future … think of today as a beautiful present wrapped in golden paper that you can unwrap, savor, and enjoy … right now, no matter where you are. Feel the **J.O.Y.**

You may wonder if this is really important to you. When you start to waver from your goals, it's important to come back to look at your answers to those five questions. That is your incentive.

Those five answers will help to reinforce your effort to take the first steps toward a healthy, happy life after 55.

More of Sara's Story

After Sara started her gratitude journal, she took more interest in steps to regain her strength. Her balance was a problem because of the surgery and the loss of core and leg strength. We began with small steps. Each week she had simple exercises to do in her kitchen. The kitchen was important for two reasons.

It gave her stable counters to lean on, and if she started to fall, she could easily grab onto a counter or a chair.

Sara started to do the balance exercises every day and write down on her calendar what she had accomplished. Her calendar became an important part of her journey to regain her health. After just four weeks, she had increased her balance from five seconds to 15 seconds on her right foot and from five seconds to 10 seconds on her left. That was a huge accomplishment for her.

There is more to Sara's story in the next chapter.

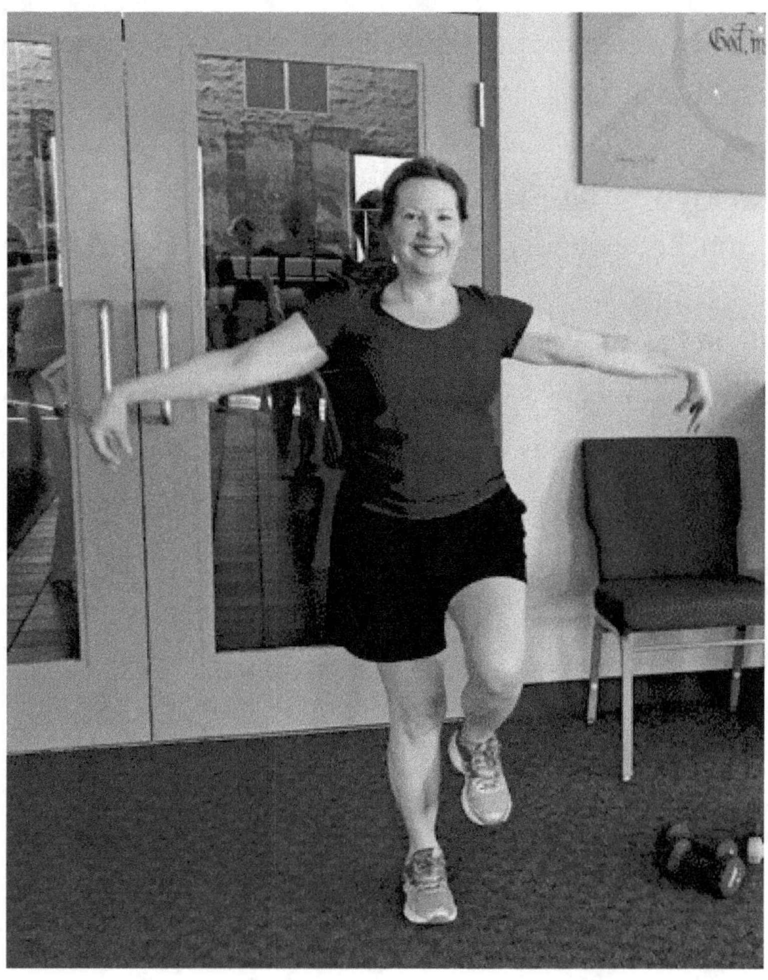

This is a participant in one of my classes. She worked on her balance every day until she could balance on one foot for 30 seconds.

You will find this exercise and others to help your balance on our Facebook page: **HealthyAfter55** for more photos and videos.

> ## What did you learn in this chapter about J.O.Y?
>
> Now is the time to begin your goal of **J.O.Y. - Just One Yes**
>
> - Take small steps, but resolve to start
>
> - Answer all five simple questions honestly and keep the answers where you can see them regularly
>
> - Take time for yourself, even if you have to put it on your calendar
>
> - Recognize how **J.O.Y.** will increase your health and happiness

The next chapter explores one of the biggest boulders that threaten your journey toward health and happiness…procrastination. Don't put it off until tomorrow…if you think that's not one of your issues, read on.

NOTE: Nothing in this book should be considered medical advice. Always consult a doctor before making any changes to your diet, medical plan, exercise routine or anything else that is important to your health. Be informed and make the best decision for your health!

Chapter 3
Stop Procrastinating

How to start your new goals...TODAY!

IN THIS CHAPTER WE WILL EXPLORE HOW procrastination prevents us from accomplishing our goals. We will have a new acronym to help set those goals and banish procrastination...at least until next week.

How can **J.O.Y.** help you stop procrastinating? It's an art that you have to practice and experience in order to feel the **J.O.Y.**

I was the princess of procrastination while I was working. You know the excuses. I work all week; I don't want to spend the weekend cleaning closets. The garage needs to be organized, but if I don't have time to organize a drawer in the kitchen, how can I find the time to clean the garage? Great excuses and I wore my princess tiara proudly. BUT when I retired, I became the *queen*.

Does that sound funny coming from someone who writes, runs, and has a busy, active life? If you are retired, you know exactly what I'm talking about.

After years of being a slave to the clock, you finally have the time to do what you want to do. The first thing you do when you retire is stop wearing a watch every day. You have *all day* to do whatever you want to do. No appointments, no kids to pick up from school or shuttle to a practice. Every day stretches out in front of you like a wonderful blank piece of paper.

And that is the problem. The blank piece of paper becomes a huge book!

I loved not having a schedule. I could do what I wanted to, when I wanted to do it. Clean the garage? Tomorrow. Except … tomorrow became next week, then next month.

The word "tomorrow" should be outlawed from the brain of every person over the age of 55. Think about how many things you've put off and decided to do tomorrow. The list never ends.

WARNING: This is going to be an important challenge. It may be more difficult than losing weight or starting to exercise. If you aren't brave enough to accept the challenge and stop procrastination in its ruby red slippers, everything else you want to do is going to pile up in a corner.

So let's go back to our goals. Procrastination never goes away. It's like the wind. You can close the door, but it will find a way through the window. You just need to figure out a way to keep it under control so it doesn't become a tornado.

As we travel on our journey to have more JOY in our lives, setting goals is important. Without goals, we wander from one shiny object to another … and accomplish nothing.

M.O.R.E is an appropriate acronym to set and achieve your goals.

M is for Move forward
O is for Original ideas
R is for Reward yourself
E is for Effort = Success

Step #1 — *Move forward.* This is where it's important to master one number … the year you were born.

When you focus on that number, you feel old, your energy evaporates, and you are frustrated because you can't do the things you did 10, 15, or 20 years ago. Procrastination just adds to that frustration.

The big celebration number that I remember when I was in my 30's was 40. Everything was black…even the frosting on the cake.

Then as Boomers reached that age and beyond, 50 became the celebration. But then an interesting thing happened. Everything wasn't black anymore. It's amazing how the Boomers even changed the attitude about birthdays, black as a celebration color and "old age".

Instead of looking at the year on your birth certificate, look at where you are right now. You can't go back, but you can learn from the past to forge a terrific future.

Mary ignored "old age" and kept moving forward.

When I started doing triathlons in my 50's, there was always this older woman, Mary, who did the short distance with her son. They were the last to cross the finish line every race.

Mary always took first place in her age group…she was the only one in her age group. I spoke to her at one race and told her she was my role model. I hoped to be competing in races for 20 years.

She laughed and said, "At 70 I'm just happy to be finishing any race upright. I've slowed down this year. I broke my hip last winter and it has taken me some time to get back on my bike.

Now, my son insists on doing the race with me. I humor him, but I could still do it by myself!"

These simple steps help you realize that the number on your birth certificate is not a barrier to an exciting life. It is a piece of paper. *Remember Mary and move forward.*

- Embrace what you have learned, the experiences you've had, and the knowledge that you can share with others.

- Use your mind to help you connect with reality so you can move forward.

- Look outside and imagine you are a butterfly floating through the air. That butterfly doesn't care how old it is. It is beautiful and can fly with ease.

- Have your children show you how to download some fun apps on your smart phone or tablet.

Step #2 — **Original ideas.** This is the time to be creative in getting things done around your house and taking the next step in a healthy life.

You think about the closet that needs to be cleaned out. You can wait until tomorrow to do it … but that thought is like a pesky mosquito. It buzzes around for a few minutes, disappears, buzzes again, and then is silent. *Inertia is the killer of accomplishment.*

What if you thought of a better way to clean it out, with the idea of giving unneeded items to a charity? Now you have a goal to clean that closet.

Yes, I finally cleaned my closet by setting a goal and giving unneeded items to charity. It worked!

- Do you have a calendar where you list all the appointments and things you have to do? Make one hour of time for yourself every day and put it on the calendar. It doesn't have to be the same time every day. Move it around so you feel comfortable doing it.

Then do it with **JOY**. Read, meditate, watch a special program on television, and go for a walk around the neighborhood. Just do something for yourself. That is an original idea to help put procrastination in the corner.

- When you brush your teeth, you probably use your dominant hand ... use some effort to try using your other hand. Start to think about what else you can do with just a minimum of effort as an original idea. Balance on one foot and then the other. Did you ever think of doing that?

- The next time you go shopping, go straight instead of turning to the right. Or turn left. It takes effort to think about doing something that isn't a habit. It's worth the effort.

The effort you take to clean that closet, think about brushing your teeth with your non-dominant hand, or taking a different route to work makes you think about what you are doing. It gives you a nudge to start thinking of ways you can incorporate a healthy lifestyle into *your* life and banish procrastination.

Step #3 — ***Reward Yourself.*** When you think of rewards, push those thoughts of ice cream and chocolate out of your mind. There are other rewards that are healthier … not that some ice cream or chocolate is out of the question, but make that a *treat* rather than a *reward*.

Just the simple act of cleaning out a drawer, working in the yard, or taking a walk can be an accomplishment when you'd rather put it off until tomorrow or next week.

Yes, it's just one more week, but you will be shocked when that day turns into a week, a month, or another year. If you just keep moving forward and accomplish small things, you will banish procrastination to a closed drawer. *For the **J.O.Y.** of it.*

Treat vs. Reward.

I would start out with a great eating and exercise plan; wholesome food, sustainable activity. At the end of the day, I would think that I deserved a reward … you guessed it … just one piece of chocolate. And then another, and another.

This was not a reward for doing something positive. It was a treat … a 500-calorie treat. That was not the reward I needed. So, I had to change my mindset.

A reward was something positive, unrelated to food, that I could feel good about at the end of the day.

The answer? I bought some cute stickers and every day that I accomplished my goals for the day, I would put a sticker on a calendar. If I didn't make my goal, no sticker on the calendar. When I collected 30 stickers, I gave myself a bigger reward … a book I had wanted to buy, a new shade of lipstick, or a new pair of running socks.

It wasn't easy to collect those 30 stickers. I had to be very honest with myself. If I was going to make the effort, it had to be based in reality. Real goals. Real rewards. Not treats.

Step #4 — ***Effort = Success.***

Think about it. One definition of effort is *a vigorous or determined attempt, either physical or mental activity that is needed to achieve something.*

One of my favorite quotes is from Winston Churchill, *"Continuous effort — not strength or intelligence — is the key to unlocking our potential."*

So now you are shaking your head and wondering what kind of effort is it going to take to be healthy. Can you dig deep and stay with this for a long time? For the rest of your life?

Remember the little test you took in the beginning of this book? Do you want to be able to play with your grandchildren? Stay independent? Live an active, vibrant life into your 80s and beyond? If your answer is yes to any of these questions, continue the effort. It will be worth it.

At 55, 65, or 75, what do you want to accomplish that you haven't done yet? Look in the mirror. Think about your life. Maybe you want to visit the Grand Canyon and be able to walk around to see the sights. Or travel to another county and be able to keep up with the rest of a tour group. The list is endless.

This is a reality check and a great way to banish procrastination.

What are you waiting for?

Sara's story continues...

Sara used her gratitude calendar and progressed with her balance. She had a better attitude and the depression was beginning to lift. She would look at me and shake my hand when I came to work with her. It was time to set some new goals.

As we set new goals, I asked Sara what activity she would like to be able to do. She smiled shyly and said, "I want to go bowling with my friends." She grabbed my hand and led me down the hall to a closet where she showed me her bowling ball and shoes. "I want to be able to lift this ball again and go bowling."

This was definitely moving forward. I had to come up with some original ideas about how to help Sara regain her strength to lift the bowling ball, lunge so she could push the ball down the alley, and focus so she could hit the pins.

Once she could do all that, it would be time to reward her for her effort.

We started with strength training for her upper body using weights and simple lunges holding onto a chair.

Then another original thought … put a cardboard box at the end of the hall to the bedroom, give her a tennis ball and have her start practicing rolling the ball into the box. She loved it.

Sara was a winner as she accomplished these goals. But she wasn't done yet …

I told you at the beginning of this chapter that I was the queen of procrastination when I retired. Writing this book was one of the things I had put off for a year. I used **MORE** goals to start and finish this project. *For the J.O.Y. of it.*

Homework for this chapter about Procrastination.

Print out this page and every week for one month, add one thing you are doing in each category to stop procrastination.

M — Move forward — Each week write down one way you moved toward a healthier lifestyle.

1.

2.

3.

4.

O — Original ideas — Each week write down one original idea to increase your health.

1.

2.

3.

4.

R — Reward yourself — Each week reward yourself with something other than food for the progress you have made

1.

2.

3.

4.

E — Effort = Success — Each week make the effort to do something healthy for yourself and then write down the effort and how it helped you be successful

1.

2.

3.

4.

NOTE: You can download a pdf or print all the homework pages at our website www.HealthyAfter55.com

What you learned in this chapter about procrastination.

*Simple steps to stop procrastination. It's all about **M.O.R.E.***

- Move forward – procrastination promotes inertia

- Original ideas – who knows what will work well for you

- Reward yourself – not with treats, but real rewards

- Effort = success – there is little success without effort

Where do we go from here?

Continue to move forward, one step at a time. Now is the time to set goals …realistic goals that you can achieve. We will show you how to do it in the next chapter.

NOTE: Nothing in this book should be considered medical advice. Always consult a doctor before making any changes to your diet, medical plan, exercise routine or anything else that is important to your health. Be informed and make the best decision for your health!

Chapter #4
Set Realistic Goals

J.O.Y. = Just One Yes is REAL

What does **JOY** have to do with setting realistic goals? *Everything*.

Think about it. When you set realistic goals, and accomplish them, **JOY** is abundant. You are ready to set more goals to have that great feeling. Positive feelings release endorphins in your brain and make you feel good. Setting goals and checking them off makes you feel great.

Sometimes the most difficult part of goal setting isn't accomplishing them …it is setting realistic goals.

How many times have you said to yourself, "I'm going to go on a strict diet and lose 10 pounds." Maybe you make it through a day, but then you are crabby and pick up pizza for dinner. So much for that goal.

Start small, keep it realistic, and keep moving forward.

When I prepared to write this book, I had a hundred different ideas about what I wanted to write about. My mind was like a hundred ping pong balls, dancing from one brilliant idea to another. I am a master of the shiny object syndrome.

Every time I read an article or talked to someone about what I could do to help them get stronger, healthier, and more positive about life, it took me down another fork in the road. Finally, I had to make a decision. It was time to set a goal.

R.E.A.L. is the acronym to set goals. I used this every day to get focused on writing this book and continue to use these goals on my own healthy lifestyle journey.

R is for Road ahead
E is for Excuses be gone
A is for Action
L is for Look forward

Step #1 — *Road Ahead*

Look at the road ahead of you. It has bumps, hills and valleys, but visualize what you are moving toward. It may be sitting comfortably on the floor playing with your grandchildren, or having renewed energy to enjoy life … or the freedom to sit in your backyard and look at the flowers that you were able to plant … all by yourself.

Enjoy those moments, whether real or imagined. That's your ultimate goal for this step of your life's journey. The goal can change when you accomplish it, but for now, it's what is important to you. The road in front of you is just one part of your life's journey.

Sometimes I think of my life as the interchange in a major city. There is so much traffic, so many exits, so little time. I have taken more wrong turns down the highway of life than I care to remember, but somehow I have ended up on a beautiful road that is my life right now.

Think about your road of life and be aware of where you are right now and where you want to go. It's not easy, but the journey can be a lot of fun.

Step #2 — *Excuses be gone*

Think about all the excuses you have for not moving forward on this extraordinary journey. Write them down. Make the list as long as possible. Really take some time to compile this list. So many "too's"…too tired, too busy, too old, too late, too lazy, too hungry, etc.

Once you've written them all down, look at this list again from the viewpoint of someone who has accomplished great things.

- Grandma Moses decided not to sit in a rocking chair and say it was too late for her to paint. She started painting at 76.

- Colonel Sanders became a major success with his Kentucky Fried Chicken at 65.

- Laura Ingalls Wilder wrote her first novel at 65 that led to the television series *Little House on the Prairie.*

This is just a few of the people who became successful after the age of 55. The list is long and impressive.

If they could follow their passion after 55, what is stopping you?

Go through your "Excuses" list and write a reason why it no longer has any meaning to you. Sounds simple, but as you move through the chapters of this book, you might get bogged down in details and think about giving up. Come back to look at the excuses that no longer have any meaning for you.

You may even laugh at a few of them and wonder why they were on your mind. And other excuses keep popping up, no matter how you try to banish them from your brain.

If you don't take control of your health now, when will you do it?

Step 3 — *Action*

Of course we need action. It's difficult to set a goal to walk a mile a day and then sit in your favorite chair and watch television. It takes effort and action to get up and accomplish that goal.

When I decided to run my first marathon, I needed to make a plan and take action to cross the finish line. After doing some research, I followed a plan for walking and running for six months before the race. Then I added nutrition steps so that I would maintain my health as I increased my exercise. Then there was strength training. I kept my eye on the goal of completing the marathon.

Every step was significant, but the most important step was taking action, taking the first step and moving forward. Every workout, every short race before the marathon mattered. It started with that very first step … and then the next … and the next. There was no magic involved.

Your goal does not have to run a marathon. It can be getting up off the floor without help or feeling more confident playing with your grandchildren. The important part is to set the goal and take that first step.

It happens when you make the effort, take action and move forward.

That brings us to the last letter.

Step 4 — *Look Forward*

You checked out the road ahead and set a goal. You banished all the excuses you could think of before starting on the journey. You set action steps. Now it's time to look forward.

When you are driving down a road, you don't just look at the stop sign in front of you. You look to the right and left, then raise your eyes to look forward toward your destination.

Whenever those excuses start to bubble up, look forward. Look at your list of excuses and think about what you can do to overcome them.

When you wonder if the journey is worth the effort, look forward.

There is always a rainbow somewhere waiting for you.

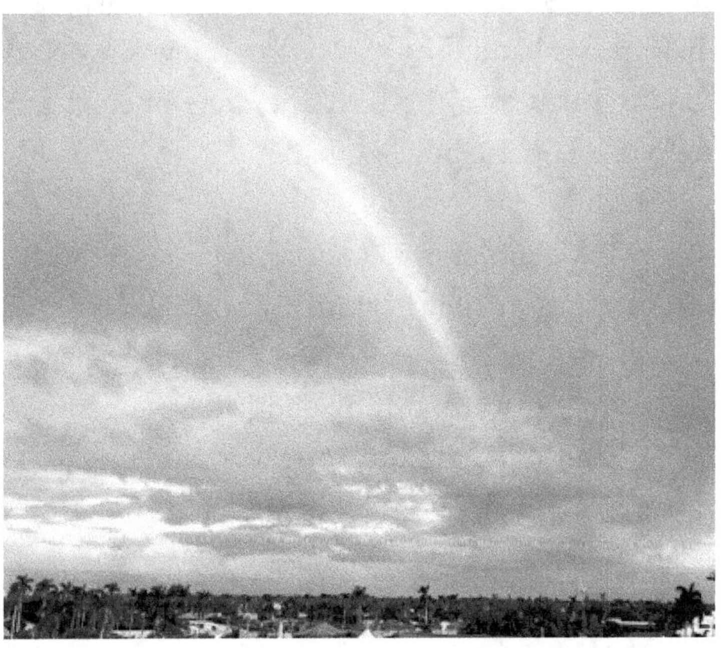

More about Sara...

We set **REAL** goals for Sara. She wanted to go bowling again with her friends. We set up realistic goals for her to regain her strength so she could lift the bowling ball. She looked forward and saw herself bowling. Her excuses were gone.

Sara started to do the lunges and became stronger. She took the action steps necessary to improve her focus. She got out that tennis ball and box and worked every day to try to roll the ball into the box.

It took her some time, but after a few weeks, when I came to her house, she greeted me at the door with a big smile and the tennis ball in her hand. She showed me how she could lunge and throw the ball into the box. Then she opened the closet door and picked up the bowling ball.

She had a twinkle in her eye. "Can we go bowling next week?" she asked. "I want to see if I can really bowl again."

Like Sara, I look forward. I think about the women I can help regain their health and vitality, to feel confident about themselves. I think about the JOY of giving back after all my years of experience.

Look forward, my friend, and you will never look back again.

NOTE: You can download a pdf or print all the homework pages at our website www.HealthyAfter55.com

Homework for this chapter on Setting Realistic Goals

Every week for the next month look at each of these sections of your R.E.A.L. goals and check them off as you accomplish them.

Goals	Week 1	Week 2	Week 3	Week 4
What did you do to move forward				
Excuses you vanquished				
Physical or mental action steps to move forward				
Goal each week				

What you learned in this chapter about realistic goals.

*You learned different ways to set realistic goals. It's all about being **R.E.A.L.***

- The road ahead of you can be bumpy and filled with challenges. Keep moving forward.

- Excuses need to be faced and overcome.

- Action is important and necessary to regain your health.

- Look forward, set realistic goals, and if you stumble, get up, dust yourself off, and continue forward.

Where do we go from here?

As you move forward with your goals toward a healthy life, attitude is important. In the next chapter you will see how attitude can help you attain the healthy goals you are setting.

NOTE: Nothing in this book should be considered medical advice. Always consult a doctor before making any changes to your diet, medical plan, exercise routine or anything else that is important to your health. Be informed and make the best decision for your health!

Chapter #5
So What?

How to change your attitude
and change your life

THIS CHAPTER IS ALL ABOUT ATTITUDE. POSITIVE, negative, or somewhere in between, everyone has an attitude. Is it really possible to change your attitude?

We've heard it before. A positive attitude will make you happier and increase your life expectancy. It's easy to say, not so easy to do.

Is a positive attitude really that important? Just go to the Internet and search for the relationship between health, wellness and attitude. You will give up before you can get through a fraction of articles and books ... and depressed by the negative influence a bad attitude can have on your overall health.

It's confusing. So much information. What's really good for you, what won't work, and what is just nonsense?

Is the same information relevant for someone in their 20's and 70's? Will it work for someone in their 50's and beyond?

Sometimes we are overwhelmed with life and just don't have the energy to make a change. We start to slip into negativity and depression. Yes, I've been there, too, and I'm usually a positive person. Sometimes a pity party just feels good. The problem starts when the pity party extends beyond an evening and into a weekend and then a week. You get the picture.

Sara's story continues…

Sara is a good example of being able to change your attitude with some hard work.

She really wanted to go bowling with her friends.

I cautioned her, "You may not be as good as you were a few years ago, but we'll figure out a way to make it work."

She smiled and said with determination, "I'm ready to try."

We went to the bowling alley on a quiet afternoon. There weren't many people bowling so there was no stress for Sara.

She was able to put her bowling shoes on, get her ball on the rack and get ready to play.

As a disclaimer, I'm not an expert bowler, but I knew enough to give her some guidelines and modifications to knock down pins.

She modified her release of the ball so she could maintain her balance, and aimed at the arrows that were close to her. She started out a little shaky, but when she got her first strike, she was thrilled! She was ready for the second and the third game.

Details on how we accomplished Sara's new goals later, but first, I am here to help you take the first steps toward a positive, healthy lifestyle. If Sara could do it, you can too.

When you think about where you are right now, you need to be realistic. Remember the acronym from the last chapter... **R.E.A.L.**

Most of your adult life you have been busy taking care of other people. Now that part of your life is slowing down. You don't feel as useful as you did when your family was younger. Where did those adult years go? Can you really begin a new chapter in your life at 55? 65? 75?

The answer is a resounding *yes*!

It won't be the same as it was when you were 25 and could just stop eating desserts and lose weight, or go for a run on the weekend and feel great the next day. There are modifications to make and ways to be smart about changing your lifestyle.

But it can be done … at any age.

Are you ready to feel healthier? Happier? Have more zest in your life?

You can begin a new chapter now, so stop thinking about what you *can't* or *don't* do anymore, and start looking at all the things you *can do*.

Let me guide you through a few simple steps to help you change your attitude. Once you do these simple steps, you will see just how important a positive attitude is to your daily life.

Remember **J.O.Y**? That's your motivation once again. *Just One Yes*. Create **JOY** every day in your life.

It's like tossing a pebble into a pond. One little pebble creates a ripple effect. Your **JOY** will spread to the people around you, the places you go, the new adventures you seek. Create **JOY** every day to make this the best chapter in your life's journey.

How do you create JOY?

- If you haven't done so already, go back and start that gratitude journal. That's how important it is to your attitude. Anything worth having and doing is worth the effort.

- Expand your journal from a single thought to multiple things. It could be listening to a favorite song that brings back wonderful memories, seeing a peaceful sunset, listening to the rain, hearing someone's laughter, thinking about a joke that made you smile, or just making it through the day.

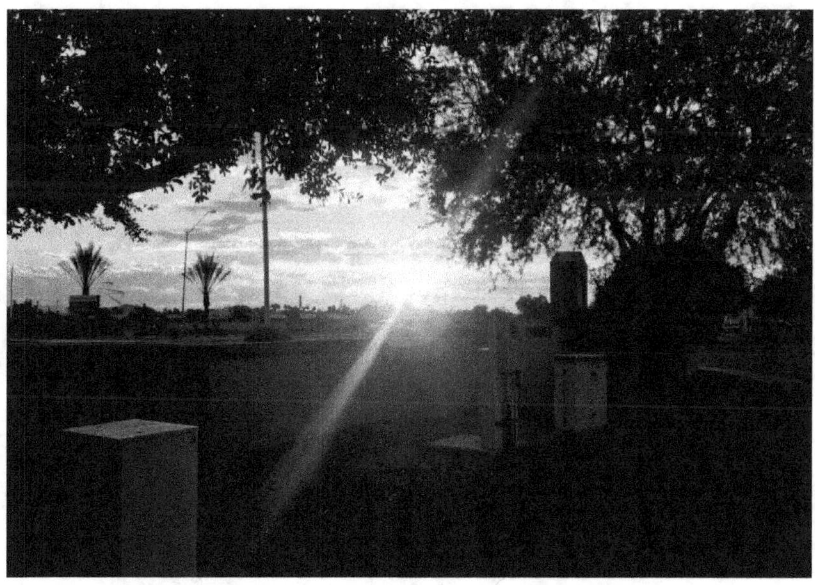

- Sometimes what you are most thankful for are the simple pleasures in your life. Think about how you feel when you come home from work to a quiet house, that first sip of cold water after cleaning the yard, a photo of your grandchild, or an email from a friend.

- Reflect on your life. Sit quietly and think about the good things that have happened to you: goals you've met, family experiences that were meaningful, people who have touched your life and the lives that you've touched.

- Awareness of your attitude is important. Be aware of your thoughts during the day. When you slide into a negative thought pattern that starts to bubble up, burst that bubble with a smile or gentle laughter. Replace it with a positive thought or feeling. Sometimes it is so much easier to be grumpy than it is to be positive.

I had a friend who could always find something negative about everything that we talked about. I could say, "I'm going to make a gourmet dinner tonight."

He would say, "I probably won't like it, so why bother?"

I would say, "I'm going to take an art class and learn to paint."

He would say, "Why would you want to do that? You can't draw a straight line with a ruler."

I think you get the point. Not a very positive relationship.

Sara's story continued ...

At first, she was hesitant to try some of the exercises that I demonstrated for her, but slowly, she began to try them and start to do them every day. She found herself getting stronger and stronger. After we went bowling, she was at the door waiting for me when I arrived, a big grin on her face. She wasn't wearing the scarf anymore; she wore a baseball cap.

She had a new goal and needed my help. More about that later.

Set a goal every morning

- Choose to do one positive thing either for yourself or someone else. Then do it. Remember the J.O.Y.

- If you get frustrated and find yourself sliding back into negativity, take a deep breath, look at your gratitude journal, and take small steps to get back on the positive road. If you need some added incentive, just turn on television and be thankful that you are not on the news.

- Every week stop for just a few minutes and think about how far you've come.

Is your attitude improved? Are you sleeping better? Are you more at peace with yourself? Getting more **JOY** out of life?

Feeling better about yourself is necessary to keep moving forward.

Your Homework for this chapter about JOY

1. If you haven't done it before, purchase a small notebook and write at least one positive thought each day.

2. Look for positive quotes and write them down. Read them every day. Post your favorites on your mirror or your refrigerator.

3. Use a calendar that has space to write and put a happy face on every day that you accomplished one positive gesture …a smile, thank you, hug, or positive gesture.

NOTE: You can download a pdf or print all the homework pages at our website www.HealthyAfter55.com

What you learned in this chapter about attitude.

The important takeaway from this chapter is to become aware of your current attitude and figure out how to minimize the negative thoughts and nurture the positive feelings for your own well-being. Think of ways you can adapt and modify your current lifestyle to increase the **JOY** and your health.

How to change your attitude.

- One word – **J.O.Y.**

- Just One Yes for yourself every day.

- It's time to be selfish. Nurture your new healthy attitude.

Now that you have a better attitude about yourself, what's next? In the next chapter you will discover just how important self-image is to attaining your healthy goals. It's time to look in the mirror and really discover the image reflected there.

NOTE: Nothing in this book should be considered medical advice. Always consult a doctor before making any changes to your diet, medical plan, exercise routine or anything else that is important to your health. Be informed and make the best decision for your health!

Chapter #6
Mirror, Mirror on the Wall

How to change the way you see yourself so you change the way others see you

WE'VE ALL LOOKED IN THAT MIRROR AND WERE shocked that it didn't shatter into a million pieces. With every passing year, it gets more and more difficult to relate that reflection with the person in your mind's eye. The mind thinks you are 30 and your body just laughs.

"A strong, positive self-image is the best possible preparation for success."

~Joyce Brothers

Think about that statement for a moment. Dr. Joyce Brothers was one of the first female psychologists to appear on television.

Many of us remember listening to her insights into being a woman in a man's world.

Self-image is more than just preparation for success in the business world. It is crucial in day-to-day thoughts and interactions with everyone.

In this chapter we will look at the reality of self-image. You will be challenged to put it into perspective …how you saw yourself 10 or 20 years ago and how you need to adjust that image for the rest of your life's journey.

It's a lot to think about, but if you really want to be healthy and enjoy this chapter of your life, it's an important goal.

Self-image is how you see yourself. Not only when you look in the mirror, but how you see yourself internally. It is not only your opinion of you physically, but what you see mentally and emotionally as well.

Do you perceive yourself to be too tall, too short, too thin, too heavy, have too much hair or not enough? Take a moment to look in the mirror and see yourself as others see you. How does it compare to how you see yourself?

This is an area that is really difficult to change. Throughout our adult lives we have been accustomed to looking at pictures of women that have been altered to make them look perfect.

If you don't look like that, you aren't as good as they are, don't deserve as much, etc., etc. Even women who are models and make their living off their looks, have things they don't like about themselves.

We've all been there. The marketers have succeeded and done their job. We spend billions of dollars trying to improve how we look on the outside. What about how we look at ourselves on the inside?

It's time to take a deep breath and do something positive for yourself.

- One important step is to think about self-image not just as the image reflected in the mirror, but also the woman behind that reflection.

- Look in the mirror and really become aware of the image that is reflected.

- Look at yourself as others see you. Do you smile, frown, look at people superficially, or really look at them? Do you see goodness in others? What do they see when they look at you? Do you see how it isn't just the physical image, but the spirit behind the image?

Remember Sara?

When I first met her, she didn't look directly at me. She wore a scarf to hide her bald head and scar. Her shoulders were rounded. She shuffled when she walked.

After we started working together, and she worked on her gratitude calendar every day, she started to change. She would laugh and tell funny stories about her family experiences. She became stronger and stood upright. She started to look at me when we talked. She stopped wearing the scarf and started wearing a baseball cap for her favorite team. She looked forward to showing me how her strength and balance improved. When she smiled, her face lit up and her eyes sparkled. Think about how her self-image had changed in just a few months.

Look in the mirror again

Think about what Sara had to endure just to get her balance back. Ask yourself, "I've done some marvelous things in my life, so why do I think I should look the same as I did 10 or 20 years ago?" When I asked myself that question, I had to laugh. I can't even remember what bothered me five years ago!

Think about how much you've changed over your adult life, the value you have from your life experiences. There is a story of strength and courage behind every line on the face that is looking back at you. Look into your eyes … see the glory and wisdom in your spirit.

Here are your goals for this important step in your life's journey. It's not easy, but the confidence and strength are so worth the effort.

The best acronym for this goal is **S.E.L.F.**

S is for See yourself as others see you
E is for Enough of the negative thoughts
L is for Love yourself
F is for Forgiveness

This may be your most difficult goal. It was for me. But once you really start to accomplish the first steps, it becomes a little easier. It's easy to relapse into old ways of thinking … you've thought the same negative thoughts about yourself for a lot of years. It's hard to break old habits.

Every time you start to think of yourself in the old, negative way, just stop, take a deep breath, and give yourself a hug, mentally or physically. You've come a long way and still have so much to accomplish on your life's journey.

Here are some simple steps to create the foundation for your improved self-image.

Step #1— ***See yourself as others see you.***

You are a vital, caring, strong, confident, loving person.

Ask a friend or someone close to you this simple question, "When you look at me, what do you see?" If you don't believe them, ask someone else. Ask your children. When you listen to them and start to believe what they are telling you about how they see you, you are going to realize that your image of yourself is very different from what other people see.

One day in my exercise class, a couple of us were talking about what we would like to change about our bodies. I patted my waist and said, "My muffin top has exploded like a can of refrigerator rolls. I need to get rid of it!"

A student in my class looked at me in disbelief. "Are you kidding? You are just a tiny little thing next to the rest of us!"

The interesting part of this story is that none of the women in the class were really big. Overweight and out of shape, yes, but not that much bigger than I was. It's all a matter of how we see ourselves.

Step #2 — ***Enough of the negative thoughts about your body.***

You are enough, just the way you are right now …you just want to improve.

In this step, take a five-minute break, sit down, close your eyes, and ask yourself, "What have I wanted to do in the last month and didn't do because I didn't think I was good enough, young enough, smart enough, energetic enough, talented enough to do it?"

That's a lot of "enough," but really think about it. What is holding you back from doing just one thing that you think you aren't good enough to do? Think about it and write it down. Post it some place where you will see it every day. Then start taking the steps necessary to make it happen.

Jessica's journey of image and health.

I led a corporate wellness challenge at a company I worked for a few years ago. One of the challenges was to start using a pedometer the company provided to everyone. We set up some goals and every week I sent out messages to encourage people to increase their steps.

One young woman, Jessica, came up to me a couple of weeks after we started the challenge. She had long hair that covered most of her face, large tinted glasses, a baggy black sweater, and baggy black pants. Her voice was very quiet as she said, "I would like to do this, but this pedometer doesn't work. Can I really lose weight just walking?"

I assured her that she could succeed if she just started to take a few more steps every day and kept a log of how many steps she walked in a week. I gave her a new pedometer, showed her how to set it, and encouraged her to check in with me every week.

She checked in every week and showed me how she was increasing her steps.

One month later, she came up to me a big smile on her face. "I lost five pounds this month, just by walking!" She laughed. "Sometimes I just have to walk around the living room at night to get my extra steps, *but it's been worth the effort.*"

There is more to her story and it all has to do with self-image.

Step #3 — ***Love yourself.***

If you don't love yourself, why should anyone else?

I always wonder why it is so difficult for us to love ourselves. We love our parents, siblings, significant others, children, pets. Why don't we feel the same love for ourselves?

Personally, I think it is because we are women. We were taught from an early age to think about other people. If we thought about ourselves, we were vain. Selfish. We needed to think about everyone else … except our own needs.

As an adult woman, we were too busy and had little time for ourselves. Now, many of those responsibilities have lessened, and we have time for ourselves, but fail to use that time in a positive way.

When you love yourself, you reflect that love to others. You've lived an amazing life. You are strong. It's time to take a step forward.

This step is easy to do, but difficult to believe.

Look in the mirror, right into your own eyes and say out loud, "I love you. You are strong. You are an amazing woman."

The first few times you do it, you will smile and you may even laugh, but take the time to do it. Do a reality check every week. Do you feel better about yourself?

Jessica's goals.

Jessica lost almost 20 pounds during the challenge, but she didn't stop there. She kept using her pedometer, counted calories, joined a gym, and lost 100 pounds in a year. Her self-image changed dramatically. She cut her hair, ditched the glasses for contacts, and wore dresses and heels to work. Her self-confidence soared. She even went back to school to get her degree.

Jessica's story is extreme, but it shows what can be accomplished by taking one step at a time and believing that you can succeed.

Step #4 — *Forgiveness.*

Forgive all the faults you see in the mirror. Move forward to a healthier, happier life. Give yourself a hug, forgive yourself and move forward on this exciting chapter of your life's journey!

If you are still having problems with loving yourself and your self-image, there are numerous self-help books available. Look for one written by a woman, for women. She understands.

Homework for this chapter on Self-Image.

Print out the chart below. Make four copies. At the end of the month compare your answers and notice the areas where you are doing well and the areas you need to focus on for improvement.

MIRROR, MIRROR – I'M THE FAIREST OF THEM ALL

Look in the mirror	Mon	Tues	Wed	Thurs	Fri	Sat	Sun
Best feature of the day							
Positive thought about myself							
Do I like how I look today?							
Love myself							

Look in the mirror	Mon	Tues	Wed	Thurs	Fri	Sat	Sun
Favorite outfit							
Be comfortable with myself							
Walk with pride							

NOTE: You can download a pdf or print all the homework pages at our website www.HealthyAfter55.com

What you learned in this chapter about self-image.

This is a big step, but when you move forward you will feel better, have more self-esteem, and have the ability to make even bigger changes in your life. Remember Jessica. She started with just one step.

- See yourself as others see you. It is a big step.

- Stop saying "I'm not good enough." You are great, and more than good enough for anything you want to accomplish.

- Love yourself first. It's time to be selfish. It may be difficult at first, but once you start, you will be an inspiration to everyone around you.

- Forgive yourself for not being the person you think you should be, or the decisions you made in the past. Start today and make decisions that will increase your health and happiness.

This is the time to be selfish and positive. You are a survivor and proud of it.

Where do we go from here? Our favorite part of the book... *move!*

NOTE: Nothing in this book should be considered medical advice. Always consult a doctor before making any changes to your diet, medical plan, exercise routine or anything else that is important to your health. Be informed and make the best decision for your health!

Chapter #7
Move It to Lose It

The Choice Is Yours

BY MOVING FOR JUST 30 MINUTES A DAY, YOU may *decrease* your chance for a stroke or heart attack … and when you do some moderate strength training you can *increase* your life expectancy.

That's motivation!

Everyone knows that exercise is good for your health. But did you know it's also good for your mood **_and_** your brain? You don't have to train for a marathon to reap the benefits. Just a 30-minute stroll is good for you.

I know, I know. Right now you are rolling your eyes and thinking of every excuse you can to just sit where you are and skip this chapter. Think about it. There are 1,440 minutes in a day. Can you set aside just 30 minutes to increase your health?

For some of you, this will be easy. You've been doing some kind of activity most of your life.

But for other people, this may be the most difficult step of all. You have excuses all lined up … too tired, too embarrassed to be seen in sweats, too busy to take the time, can't afford a gym membership, it's just not worth the effort. *It is worth the effort.*

In this chapter, I will show you some simple steps to get started. You don't even need to take one step outside your house. You can do many of these things in the comfort and privacy of your own living room.

The important thing to remember is that you are doing this for *your* health. It really doesn't matter what anyone else thinks about it.

S.T.E.P. is the logical acronym for this goal. Get ready to move forward, one step at a time.

S is for Start
T is for Take your time
E is for Effort
P is for Purpose

Step #1 — Start moving.

This is the hardest part. Just take that first step and build slowly. Don't do what I did. I tried to run before I could walk a mile and signed up for a 5k (3.1 miles) when I hadn't walked that far in five years.

Here is an easy way to get started in your own home. Sit on a solid chair (kitchen or dining room chair) and without using your hands, stand up. Sit down again, count to 5, and stand up again. Focus on using your thighs and your core to sit and stand. Practice this until you can do it during an entire commercial on television. When you can do it through one commercial, try doing it through a second commercial, until you can do it through all the commercials in a half hour show.

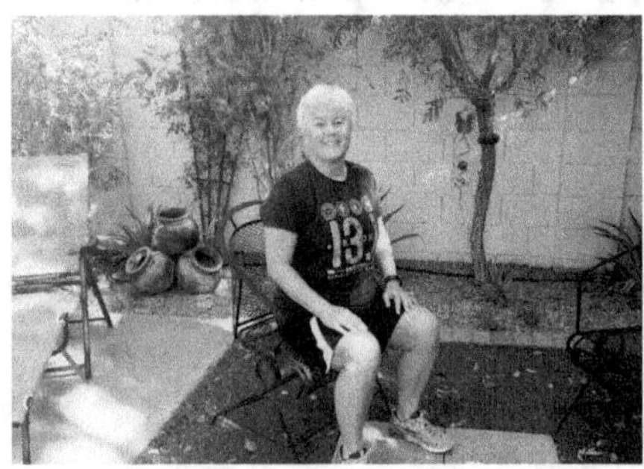 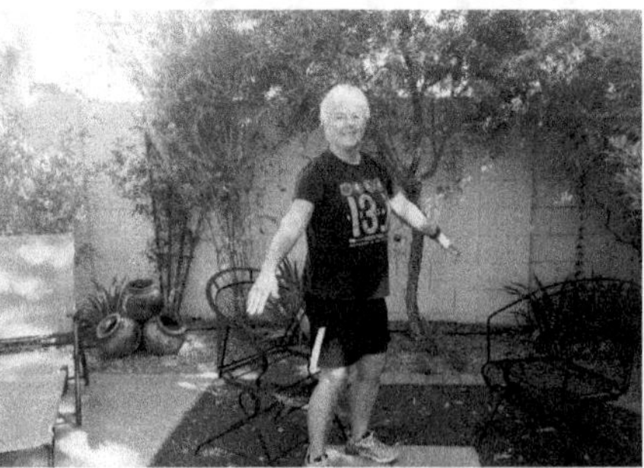

Step #2 — *Take your time.*

If your goal is to ultimately run a local race or lose 20 pounds, start with walking around the block or losing one pound. Look at the ultimate goal realistically. You want to keep moving forward as much as possible.

Joanne's story.

One of the ladies I worked with when I was a personal trainer, Joanne, had a difficult time doing any of the things I suggested during the week when we didn't meet.

At one of our sessions I had her tell me about some of the things she loved to do and what motivated her to do them. She loved to quilt and showed me photos of beautiful quilts she had created. I suggested that she use her calendar, set a goal each day to complete one of exercises I suggested for her, and when she accomplished that goal, she could begin quilting.

I didn't realize what an exciting event this would become. Joanne not only started setting and accomplishing her exercise goals, but she made several beautiful placemats, and gave two of them to me when she lost ten pounds. That was a great win-win for both of us.

Step #3 — *Effort*

This can be the hardest part of any lifestyle change. It won't be easy. You will fall off the wagon and have to crawl back on, but the effort is worth the quality of life that you are creating for yourself. No one can do it for you. This is something that only you can do.

- This is where you want to take a deep breath, close your eyes, and remember when you started reading this book. You first pictured in your mind's eye the inability to get off the floor to save your grandchild who ran out the door. Then you pictured yourself being capable of getting up and reaching them before any harm could be done. That took effort and you need to keep that feeling to maintain the effort.

- A fun way to track your effort is to use your calendar again.

- Buy some fun stickers and put one on your calendar every day you do something physical. It could be gardening, cleaning the house, taking a walk in the neighborhood, parking your car a little farther away from the store, playing with your children, taking a pet for a walk, or dancing around the house. Anything physical. When you make it something you like to do, you will be more likely to continue doing it.

Step #4 — ***Purpose.***

Remind yourself of the reasons you want to do this for not only yourself, but also for your loved ones. Pull out the list of reasons why it's important for you to increase the quality of your life. Add to that list as you think of more reasons why your health is a priority.

This was an important step for me. One day I just didn't have the energy to do anything physical. I sat and read a book, ate junk food, and had a margarita instead of water. I tossed and turned all night, woke up even more lethargic than I had been the day before. That day and night turned into a week.

That's when I woke up on a Saturday morning, looked at my reasons for wanting to be healthy, evaluated how I felt after doing nothing positive for five days, and realized how important my health was to my happiness and how much it mattered to my family.

Have you ever thought or said…

"It's too hot (or cold) to go outside. There isn't anything I can do in the house."

"I don't like to exercise."

"I don't want to go to an expensive gym."

"I'm too embarrassed to exercise in front of anyone."

"I don't have workout clothes."

"I can't find my shoes."

"I don't have any equipment."

"I'm too old, too overweight, too sore."

"I'd rather watch my favorite TV show."

Your purpose for being healthy is what will keep you motivated and moving toward a healthier lifestyle.

No more excuses! Here are some simple exercises that anyone can do at home.

NOTE: *Please! If anything hurts, don't do it! Always check with your health care professional before starting any exercise program or trying anything new.*

- Turn on your radio or music on your smart phone. Find something that you like, that makes you think about something fun when you were young. Start moving to the music (if your neighbors see you, so much the better!)

- Don't want to dance? Pretend you are the conductor and wave your arms.

- Do you have a garden or plants that need watering and trimming? Bending over to pull out weeds is great exercise. Just make sure to "hinge" from your hips, keep your back flat and your head in line with your back. It will take the pressure off your lower back. Please visit my Facebook page: **HealthyAfter55** for a video on an easy way to pick something up off the floor or ground.

- Walk around a room or your yard while alternating knee lifts with each step, raising the opposite arm at the same time. When you can do it easily, try doing it raising your arm and leg on the same side.

- Sit on a chair with both feet on the floor, slowly raise one foot about 6 inches off the floor and hold it to the count of 10. Slowly put it back on the floor. Repeat 10 times. Switch to the other leg.

- Park next to the shopping cart drop off when you go grocery shopping. Walk down every aisle at the store before checking out. You will be surprised at how many minutes you are active.

More about Jessica.

By the time we did another wellness challenge a year after she first started counting her steps, she had lost over 100 pounds.

She not only had more confidence, but she was happier and healthier! After she went back to school to get her degree, she was ready to move on. She landed a job she had dreamed about for a long time and moved across the country to start a new life.

We stayed in touch and Jessica has continued to set more goals for herself. She completed her first marathon just a few months ago and sent me a photo of herself, a big smile on her face as she held up her medal after finishing the race.

Jessica achieved health and happiness ... *one step at a time.*

Resistance training is a good way to strengthen your muscles.

These are easy exercises you can do with a bath towel while watching TV. You can see demonstrations of these exercises on our Facebook page: **HealthyAfter55** for more photos and videos.

- Grasp one end of your bath towel with your left hand and wrap the towel around your back. Grasp the other end of the towel with your right hand. Pull on the towel with both hands while standing tall. Hold it for a count of 10. Relax and do it again. Repeat it 5 times; gradually increase the amount of time you can keep the resistance on the towel. This strengthens your core, back, grip, fingers and wrists.

- Sit down on a chair or the floor, grasp the towel in both hands and slide it under your right foot. Keep your leg straight and pull on the towel. Do the same thing with your left leg. When this is easy to do, try raising your leg slightly when you pull on the towel.

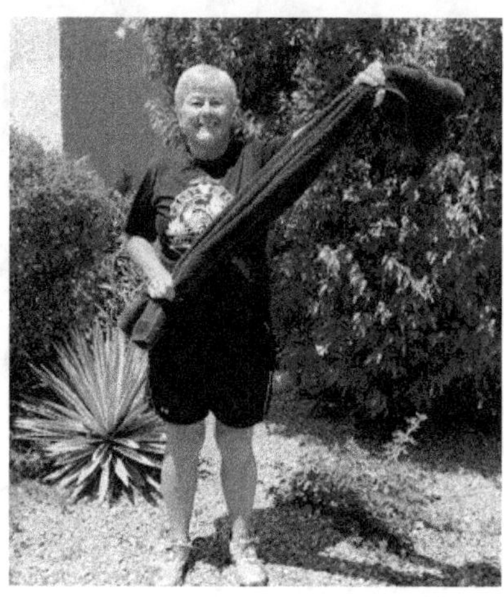

- Grasp the ends of the towel with your hands and try to pull the towel apart. First raise your right hand and pull, then your left hand. This is a great exercise to strengthen your grip, wrists and arms without putting too much pressure on your joints.

No weights for strength training? No problem.

- You can do this exercise when you are at the park watching your children or grandchildren play a sport. Use a couple of water bottles (good way to remember to drink water). When they are empty, fill them with small stones or sand to add a little weight. (Unopened soup cans also work when you do these exercises at home.

- Hold one bottle in each hand, palms up. Slowly curl one arm up, keeping your elbow at your side. Hold it for a count of 5 and then slowly return your hand to your side. Repeat this 5 times with one arm and then switch to the other arm. When you can do it easily, do both arms at the same time.

- Hold one bottle in your right hand, your arm at your side. Push your hand back until you can feel the tension in the back of your upper arm. Hold it for a count of 5 and return your arm to the start. Repeat 5 times and then do the same thing with your left arm.

- Take deep breaths to help you relax. Try it the next time you feel stressed. Sit or stand, take a deep breath in through your nose, count to 5, and exhale through your mouth. Just do this 2 or 3 times and then relax.

For videos of these exercises and additional easy exercises you can do at home, please visit my Facebook page: **HealthyAfter55** for more photos and videos.

Move more for a healthier __you__.

No more excuses.

Homework for this chapter on Exercise.

If you are able, purchase an inexpensive pedometer (available in the Sporting Goods Department at most stores) or use your smartphone with an app (good if you keep your phone in your pocket all day). See how many steps you currently average every day.

- Increase that number just a little bit each day and then look at your totals for the week.

- Keep track and give yourself a pat on the back for a job well done when you consistently increase that number!

- Each day write down what exercise you did and the effort you put into it on a scale of 1–5

- Scale for effort
  - 1 = no effort
  - 2 = not breathing hard
  - 3 = starting to breath hard, a little sweaty
  - 4 = working up a sweat, breathing hard
  - 5 = difficult to finish, but you did it!

	Mon	Tues	Wed	Thurs	Fri	Sat	Sun
Week 1							
Week 2							
Week 3							
Week 4							

NOTE: You can download a pdf or print all the homework pages at our website www.HealthyAfter55.com

What you learned in this chapter about movement.

You learned that it is important to take that first step toward physical exercise. You can do all the other things necessary for good health, but if you neglect movement, you set yourself up for failure.

- Start with one step and keep moving forward

- Take your time as you make this important lifestyle change

- Effort is important to maintain your new exercise goals

- Purpose will keep you focused as you remember the reason you want to be healthy

Now that you are moving more … what's next? The chapter that you've been waiting for … food!, Food and diet are both four-letter words but have a different meaning to each of us. We will explore some ways for you to find the best way to eat healthy and continue toward your healthy goals.

NOTE: Nothing in this book should be considered medical advice. Always consult a doctor before making any changes to your diet, medical plan, exercise routine or anything else that is important to your health. Be informed and make the best decision for your health!

Chapter #8
DIET is a Four Letter Word

Eating healthy foods can increase your life expectancy

OF COURSE, YOU PROBABLY *KNEW* THAT, BUT *doing* it is more difficult to accomplish. In fact, it is one of the most challenging steps you will take. If you were looking through the book, saw the chapter on diet, and decided to jump ahead to this chapter, you will be disappointed.

If you expected a miracle announcement to help you lose weight while eating whatever you want to eat …it's not going to happen.

Diet really is a four letter word. You are bombarded with ads regarding what to eat and how to lose weight every day. Some make sense but others are difficult to follow for more than a week or two.

This is one of my favorite quotes regarding diets and losing weight.

"In two decades I've lost a total of 789 pounds. I should be hanging from a charm bracelet."

~ Erma Bombeck

If you are like me, you've tried so many different weight loss programs, you can't even remember all of them. One of my more memorable weight loss experiments was a seminar that involved hypnosis to turn off the desire for food. My friend and I went out for pizza and glass of wine when the seminar ended.

Many of us have lived the "food fight" all of our lives! You start another diet with high hopes; lose a couple of pounds, and then life gets in the way…AGAIN! You gain it back plus a few more pounds and inches. And it gets more difficult with each passing year.

Have you ever said …

"Eating is such a pleasure."

"Why should I bother changing my eating habits now?

"I'm too old to change what I eat."

"It won't make any difference."

Just like every other positive step you take for a healthier, happier life, this will be a challenge and take effort…but, it is never too late to start eating for a healthy life.

This chapter is going to give you some tips to get started on a healthy journey. You may decide you are fine just the way you are right now, but there is always room for improvement.

It makes sense that your goals for healthy eating would be **F.O.O.D.**

F is for *Follow a healthy eating plan*
O is for *Ounces of water*
O is for *Out of sight, out of mind*
D is for *Don't dwell on mistakes*

Step #1 — ***Follow a healthy eating plan***.

- This is an important part of your plan for a healthier, happier life. Find a qualified nutritionist who understands your health issues and can help you find an eating plan that will work for years to come, not just a few weeks.

- Find an app for your smart phone to help you track what you eat every day. There are plenty of apps available. Find one that is motivating and will keep you focused on your goal.

- If you have any health issues, make sure to check with your healthcare professional before starting any eating plan. This is for your long-term health, not a quick fix.

Step #2 — *Ounces of water — drink more.*

- Figure out how much water you need to drink to stay hydrated. There are many articles on the Internet to figure out how much you need to drink every day.

- A good way to start is with a glass of water every time you eat something. It not only makes you aware that you are putting food into your mouth, but it helps to increase your water intake.

- Again, check with your healthcare professional to make sure you are drinking the correct amount of water.

Step #3 — *Out of sight, out of mind.*

- The nutritionist can help guide you to make the best decisions for your health and your body.

- Read the labels. If it has ingredients that aren't good for you, toss it out. If you just can't bring yourself to throw it out, give it to a food bank or homeless shelter. You can't eat what you don't see.

- Be wary of those television commercials in the evening. Just when you think you've conquered your eating for the day, you may be tempted by those commercials. Turn off television and read a book or take a walk.

Step #4 — ***Don't dwell on mistakes***.

- If you eat something you know isn't good for you, don't dwell on it.

- Think about why you ate it, acknowledge that you ate something that wasn't the best for your health, and move on.

- Don't use it as an excuse to eat everything in sight.

- Take a deep breath, drink a glass of water, and move forward.

It's never too late to eat healthy!

Change just a little at a time. Every goal starts with just one step. Changing your eating habits can seem overwhelming, but it doesn't need to be.

Vanessa's story

When I taught spin classes, a lady came to class one day in a sweat shirt and sweat pants. She stared at the bike and I could tell she was ready to run out the door. I greeted her and shook her hand. Vanessa had a strong handshake and a look of desperation on her face.

She told me in a quiet voice that she wanted to have a baby, but the doctor said she needed to lose at least 50 pounds to increase her odds of getting pregnant and having a healthy baby. Now, that was a goal! She said she had talked to the nutritionist at the doctor's office and she had suggested that Vanessa start exercising as well as eating the well-balanced diet that had been given to her.

I encouraged Vanessa to start doing the spin class because it would take the stress off her joints while she lost weight and would give her a good cardio workout. Little did she know just how good the workout would be!

After getting the bike set up for her, she climbed on and held on as if her life depended on it. I told her that she could stop after ten minutes. Everyone else in the class would understand because they had all been there at one time. She shook her head. "I can ride a bike for an hour. No problem." Vanessa lasted 15 minutes.

The important part is that Vanessa came back to class three times a week, increased her time in class every week until she made it through the whole class …and stopped wearing sweats.

More of Vanessa's story later …

You don't need to eat kale for breakfast every day to live a healthy life …but it will take effort on your part. It's all about awareness and making positive decisions.

- Do your research. Think about what worked for you in the past and might work again.

- Consult with a nutritionist to make a plan for the foods that are best for you and your lifestyle …talk to your health care professional about any health concerns and what type of eating plan is best for you. Ask friends for a referral. Find out about their background. If they've never struggled with a weight issue, it may be difficult for them to understand your challenges. If they have had weight issues, they will understand what you need to do and help you make the changes. I would also suggest that you find someone who is over the age of 40. They understand the changes to your body as you get a little older, and how difficult it is to just maintain your weight, let alone lose some pounds.

- Find healthy foods that you like and try new recipes … or old recipes you haven't made in a long time. You can find *something* that you like and is good for you.

- Pull out one of those old diet books. What worked for you?

- Do you have a blender? Make your own smoothie, be creative. Experiment with different fruit and veggies. There are so many different kinds of "milk"…almond, cashew, unsweetened, sweetened, vanilla, dark chocolate. Find something you like and your stomach tolerates.

- Include fruit and vegetables, nuts and beans, lean meat, and healthy oils in your meals. Variety is the key to get all the nutrients you need so you age in a healthy manner.

- Is there a Farmer's Market in your community? It's a great place to buy seasonal fresh fruits and veggies. It saves you money, supports local farmers, and gives you a variety of fresh food to eat.

- If you really love that glass of wine with dinner or that bowl of ice cream, don't banish it forever. Just be aware of when and how much you are consuming … eating a pint of ice cream at one time is seldom a great idea. I love ice cream and anything with chocolate in it. I started to buy the single serving ice cream cups and over time, that helped to shave lots of empty calories from my eating plan. I still had the occasional treat, but not so many calories consumed.

- Eat fresh whenever possible … seasonal fruits and vegetables are budget-friendly and make for a good variety. I like to make chili in the winter, but don't want to eat it all week. I freeze it in individual containers and pull one out when I don't feel like cooking.

- Have healthy snacks. An apple and a tablespoon of nut butter (cashew or almond are my favorites) is an easy snack that is healthy and tasty.

- Eat healthy meals at home. Then when you go out to eat indulge in a favorite food. You can always bring half of it home and enjoy it the next day.

More about Vanessa…

Vanessa took that first step by trying spin class and following the healthy eating plan suggested by the nutritionist. In five months, Vanessa had accomplished her goal of losing 50 pounds and was determined to lose more weight.

She bought cycling shorts and started to wear sleeveless workout shirts. She asked if I had a training plan to go from walking to running. Of course I did!

A couple of months later, Vanessa asked if she could join me for a 10k race. We did the race together. I don't know who was more thrilled when we crossed the finish line. She gave me a big hug and said she had not only lost another ten pounds, but she was pregnant!

One step at a time …

Your homework for this chapter.

Complete each chart every week. If you didn't complete an item, put a zero. At the end of the week add up your numbers.

Yes   No

☐   ☐   Have a healthy eating plan to follow this week.

☐   ☐   Eating more fruits and veggies than I did last week.

☐   ☐   Drank at least 8 glasses of water this week.

☐   ☐   Read labels and put high sugar foods in the back of the cupboard.

☐   ☐   Avoided sugar at least once a day.

☐   ☐   Used real food instead of process food at least once a day.

☐   ☐   Tracked my calories and exercise.

Totals

Yes   No

☐   ☐   Have a healthy eating plan to follow this week.

☐   ☐   Eating more fruits and veggies than I did last week.

☐   ☐   Drank at least 8 glasses of water this week.

☐   ☐   Read labels and put high sugar foods in the back of the cupboard.

☐   ☐   Avoided sugar at least once a day.

☐   ☐   Used real food instead of process food at least once a day.

☐   ☐   Tracked my calories and exercise.

Totals

Yes   No

☐   ☐   Have a healthy eating plan to follow this week.

☐   ☐   Eating more fruits and veggies than I did last week.

☐   ☐   Drank at least 8 glasses of water this week.

☐   ☐   Read labels and put high sugar foods in the back of the cupboard.

☐   ☐   Avoided sugar at least once a day.

☐   ☐   Used real food instead of process food at least once a day.

☐   ☐   Tracked my calories and exercise.

Totals

Yes   No

☐ ☐ Have a healthy eating plan to follow this week.

☐ ☐ Eating more fruits and veggies than I did last week.

☐ ☐ Drank at least 8 glasses of water this week.

☐ ☐ Read labels and put high sugar foods in the back of the cupboard.

☐ ☐ Avoided sugar at least once a day.

☐ ☐ Used real food instead of process food at least once a day.

☐ ☐ Tracked my calories and exercise.

Totals

Score for each week:

7 YES! = You are a super star and well on your way to being healthy after 55

5–6 YES! = You are moving forward and making the effort

3–4 YES! = It's time to try harder and accept the challenge of being healthy after 55

0–2 YES! = Evaluate why it is difficult for you to follow these simple guidelines and resolve to do better next week

NOTE: You can download a pdf or print all the homework pages at our website www.HealthyAfter55.com

> ## What you learned in this chapter about healthy eating.
>
> You learned that diet is more than a four-letter word. A healthy eating plan is critical for a healthy lifestyle.
>
> - Follow a healthy eating plan that works for you
>
> - The amount of water you drink every day is important – count the ounces
>
> - Out of sight, out of mind - move the food that is not so healthy to the back of the cupboard
>
> - Don't dwell on mistakes that you may make along the way, learn from them and move on

What's next? This is the fun part … something you do all the time, but don't realize it's important for your health. Take a guess before going to the next page.

NOTE: Nothing in this book should be considered medical advice. Always consult a doctor before making any changes to your diet, medical plan, exercise routine or anything else that is important to your health. Be informed and make the best decision for your health!

Chapter #9
Talk, Talk, Talk

Socialization is just as important as healthy eating and exercise for your total well-being.

STUDIES HAVE SHOWN THAT PEOPLE WHO ARE isolated tend to age quicker than those who stay engaged with friends and relatives.

Socializing is defined as the *activity of mixing socially with others.* It should not be confused with the definition of social media which is *websites and applications that enable users to create and share content to participate in social networking.*

Socialization is much than just scrolling through Facebook and "liking" a post. There are many positive things about social media. It's a great way to stay in touch with family and friends.

This may be one of the easier steps you take toward your goal of a healthier life…or it may be another challenge. Everyone is different.

You may nod your head and think that you already do enough socializing so you can skip this chapter.

Face-to-face interaction and actually talking to people can be one of the most important steps you take for a healthier, happier life.

If you are still working, you may think you don't need to read this chapter because you are talking to people all day and need a break. That may be true, but you need to be aware of the *quality* of your interaction with people.

Do you spend most of your time with a headset on talking on the telephone? When you speak to the people around you, do you smile and laugh or does everyone complain? Does everyone treat each other with respect? The quality of your interaction each day can have a huge impact on your health.

Try for a balance of positive, happy interactions with the normal work interactions. It may not be easy, but it will help you lead a healthier, happier life.

If you are retired, this chapter is especially important. Once you are out of the work force, you may have limited interaction with other people. It takes effort to get out of the house and talk to people. It's much easier to talk to your television or your computer, but the reaction you get is not the same.

It makes sense that your goal for this chapter is **T.A.L.K.**

T is for Talk to people
A is for Awareness
L is for Like
K is for Know

Step #1 — *Talk to people*

Face-to-face speaking with someone else is quality socialization.

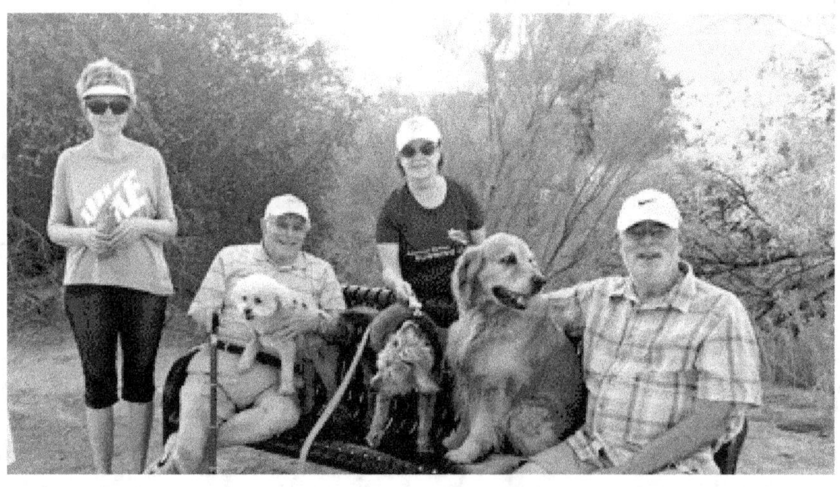

These friends meet at the park every day to walk their dogs, and most importantly, talk to each other!

I remember when I would go shopping with my mother and she would talk to the clerk in the store, the teller at the bank, just about everyone. Drove me crazy! Then I realized that after she retired, she was home alone with just her cat to talk to and he didn't respond unless he was hungry. She needed the social interaction.

I relaxed and smiled as she held up the line in the grocery store while she talked to the clerk. And yes, I've become my mother. Now, I get to drive my kids crazy.

Step #2 — Awareness of what's going on around you.

- If you see someone who needs a smile, be the one to share. How much effort does that take? Be aware of how often you stay at home by yourself and how many hours you spend without saying a word.

- Join a book club. You will stimulate your brain **_and_** increase your social activity. Check your local library to see if they have any book clubs. If not, start one with a few of your friends.

- Think about what interests you and look for ways to do it! How about going to an exercise class, having fun, **_and_** socializing?

- Really listen when someone is speaking to you. Look at their face, their eyes. Concentrate on what they are saying. It's all about awareness.

Step #3 — ***Like people, really like them … not just hit a button on social media sites.***

- Show people that you like them rather than just tolerating them. Like their pets. Tell your friends how much you like doing things with them.

- Use social media to your advantage. Comment on posts and write why you like them. Avoid negative posts that make you depressed or angry.

- Text messages to your friends and family. Learn how to post photos and use fun emoji's. If you don't know how to do something, ask a family member or friend. They will be happy to help you.

Step #4 — ***Know how important it is to interact with others.***

- Take stock of how to improve your interaction with other people.

- If you know you've been avoiding friends or family because it's just too much effort, then make time to figure out how to improve the relationships. Be honest. You know what needs improving. Now is the time to do it.

- If you are unable to get out of the house, invite a friend over for a cup of coffee or tea. Talk about memories as well as what's going on in the local news right now. Stay engaged.

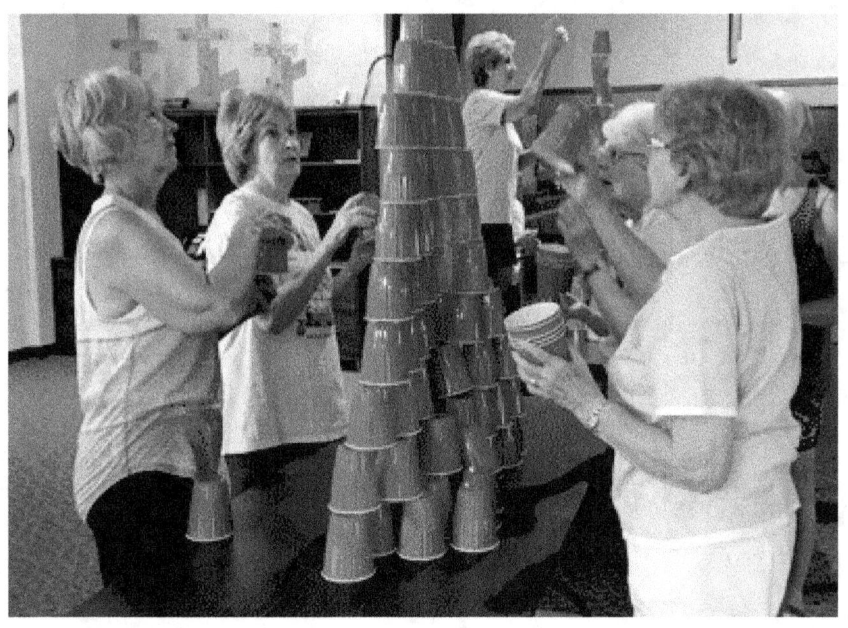

These ladies are using their creative minds, socializing, and best of all ...having fun!

NOTE: The next time you have a family gathering, try this game. See how tall a pyramid of red cups your guests can make in one or two minutes.

Your homework for this chapter on Socialization.

Every day, do just one of the following activities to increase your socialization.

______ Just once a day, talk to someone!

______ If you are unable to get out of the house, invite a friend over for a cup of coffee or tea. Talk about memories as well as what's going on in the local news right now. Stay engaged.

______ If you are able to get out of the house, meet friends for breakfast, attend church services, volunteer! One of the ladies in my exercise class is 84 and still volunteers at the local library!

______ Join a book club. You will stimulate your brain ***and*** increase your social activity. Check your local library to see if they have any book clubs.

______ Do you like to play cards? Join a card club …or start one yourself with a few of your friends.

______ Volunteer at a school to help children read.

______ If you are still working, talk to a coworker you don't know very well. Really listen when they speak to you. Look at their face, their eyes. Concentrate on what they are saying.

_____Take your pet to the park and talk to the other pet owners.

_____ Renew an old acquaintance.

_____ Make an on-going appointment with a friend to walk every week.

Week 1   Week 2   Week 3   Week 4

_______   _______   _______   _______

Each week

Completed 6–7 opportunities to socialize = Superstar! Socialization comes easy to you. Keep up the good work.

Completed 4–5 opportunities to socialize = You are doing okay. Try to increase your number each week.

Completed 2–3 opportunities to socialize each week = Not very social. Take some time to figure out what you can do to increase your number each week.

Completed 0–1 opportunities to socialize each week = INTROVERT! You need to make the effort to socialize. This is important to your health and wellness. Make the time to try at least two opportunities next week.

NOTE: You can download a pdf or print all the homework pages at our website www.HealthyAfter55.com

What you learned in this chapter about socialization.

You learned the importance of socialization and how it relates to your goal of increased health and happiness. It's all about *T.A.L.K.*

- Talk to people and really listen to them

- Have an awareness of the people around you and reach out to them

- Like more than just social media; genuinely like the people around you

- Know what works for you, but step out of your comfort zone occasionally

Stay connected with the outside world, your family, friends, and neighbors. **J.O.Y.** can be found everywhere.

Where do we go from here?

You are close to completing the important first steps of your journey to regain and maintain your health and happiness after 55. Now, put it all together.

NOTE: Nothing in this book should be considered medical advice. Always consult a doctor before making any changes to your diet, medical plan, exercise routine or anything else that is important to your health. Be informed and make the best decision for your health!

Chapter #10
What's Next?

You've made great progress on your journey toward health and happiness after 55 ... but there is more work to do!

WE TALKED ABOUT THE WORD "TOMORROW" AND the need to banish it when you are setting goals and doing things that improve your health.

Let's think about that a little more. Think about tomorrow. Look back at the road you've traveled and where you want to go.

Look back to your goals. As you travel on your journey to have more **JOY** in your life, become more at peace with your life, and discover what **"MORE"** means to you personally.

So here is your last set of goals for this book. **M.O.V.E.** — It means more than putting one foot in front of the other.

M is for Move forward
O is for Organize your life
V is for Value what you've already done
E is for Evolve into a healthy person

Do it with **J.O.Y.**

Step #1 — ***Continue to move forward with your health and with your life's journey.***

Take the steps necessary to regain your health and then maintain it as you continue on your life's journey. You have some great years ahead of you. Do you want to sit in a chair and think about the life you might have had? Do you want to be an observer or a participant in your life?

Step #2 — ***Organize your life.***

Not just cleaning the drawers or cupboards, but thinking about where you want this healthy life to take you. Think about your future, the skills you have, what you want to accomplish in the next year, five years, ten years. Where you want to live, what legacy you want to leave, the steps you need to take to maintain your health and independence.

Step #3 — ***Value what you've accomplished in your life.***

You can't put a price tag on them, but you can value the skills, the memories, the strong person you've become. If you are strong emotionally and mentally, it's time to be strong physically as well.

Step #4 — ***Evolve and develop into the healthy person you were meant to be.***

All these years you've been helping others. Now it's time to be selfish. Think about where you want to be, how important your health is to you and those around you, and then do something about it. Evolve into the person you want to be.

Those are your goals for this chapter and for every chapter of your life that is ahead of you. Look forward with excitement, expectancy, and a vibrant outlook. You've accomplished so much in the last 50+ years. Think of what you can accomplish in the next 50!

Homework for this chapter to Put It All Together.

Before we set more goals, take some time to sit and answer these questions. Make them personal. This is all about you.

1. If you are working, do you like your job? Are you counting the weeks, days, hours, until you can retire? Given the chance, what would you rather be doing right now?

2. Assess your job skills and think about what you've accomplished that you could use in another line of work or in a different company. If you are happy where you are, think about adding some new skills that will make you more valuable. Think outside the box. Many skills can transfer to jobs you never thought about before.

3. Are you living where you want to spend the rest of your life? This is a tough question. Maybe you've lived in the same community or area of the country for your entire life, your family is still there, and you want to stay right where you are. Then one of your children moves across the state or a thousand miles away and takes your only grandchild with them. Is your original answer still the same? Maybe you had a really brutal winter of snow and cold. You just shoveled the sidewalk in April and couldn't find the daffodils. Is your answer still the same? Stay open to change. Explore new and different locations.

What does this have to do with being healthy after 55? It's all about choices, being open to new adventures, and facing this chapter of your life's journey with excitement.

NOTE: You can download a pdf or print all the homework pages at our website www.HealthyAfter55.com

What you learned in this book

Most importantly, you learned that it isn't easy to lead a healthy life after 55. It takes courage and strength to take that first step, but as you move forward, you will have more energy, stronger independence, increased self-esteem, and you will be ready for this exciting part of your life's journey.

This is where the acronyms for this book are really important. You may not remember everything you read, but you can remember these simple goals.

J.O.Y = Just One Yes

M.O.R.E = Move, Organize, Reward, Effort

R.E.A.L = Road, Excuses, Action, Look Forward

S.E.L.F = See Yourself, Enough, Love, Forgiveness

S.T.E.P = Start, Take Your Time, Effort, Purpose

F.O.O.D = Follow Healthy Plan, Ounces of Water, Out of Sight, Don't Dwell

T.A.L.K = Talk to People, Awareness, Like, Know

M.O.V.E = Move Forward, Organize your Life, Value, Evolve

But wait … there's more …

This is just the beginning of living your best life … your life after 55.

Save the homework that you did in each chapter. Date them and print another set when you've completed them.

When you start the next set of homework, set your goals a little higher. Accomplish more. Challenge yourself.

Then read the next three books in this series as we go into more depth with the ideas presented here.

There will be more goals to set, more stories to tell, and some unique ways to increase your health and happiness that you may not have thought about before.

You will hear more about Sara and the new goals she has set for herself.

And learn what happened to Vanessa's goals after she had her baby.

NOTE: Nothing in this book should be considered medical advice. Always consult a doctor before making any changes to your diet, medical plan, exercise routine or anything else that is important to your health. Be informed and make the best decision for your health!

About the Author

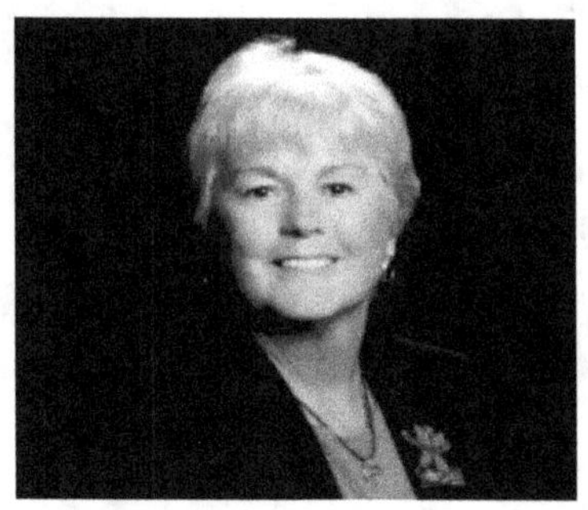

JULIE LUEDTKE is an American Council on Exercise certified personal trainer and certified by National Institute of Health Science to train older adults. She lives in Phoenix, Arizona where she teaches exercise classes for older adults. She lives what she teaches. At 73, she still does half marathons, hikes, bikes and writes. Julie loves educating and inspiring adults to live life to the fullest … no matter what their birth certificate says.

See videos for more detailed instructions presented here on her Facebook page, Healthy After 55.

One Last Thing...

If you enjoyed this book or found it useful I'd be very grateful if you'd post a short review on Amazon. Your support really does make a difference. I read all the reviews personally so I can get your feedback and make this book even better.

Thanks again for your support!

NOTE: Nothing in this book should be considered medical advice. Always consult a doctor before making any changes to your diet, medical plan, exercise routine or anything else that is important to your health. Be informed and make the best decision for your health.

www.ingramcontent.com/pod-product-compliance
Lightning Source LLC
Chambersburg PA
CBHW061349250726
48657CB00004B/1408